the orthomolecular approach to

learning disabilities

allan cott, m.d.

academic therapy publications
novato, california

Academic Therapy Publications
20 Commercial Boulevard
Novato, California 94947

Books, tests, and materials
for and about the learning disabled

Library of Congress Cataloging in Publication data

Cott, Allan, 1910 -
  The orthomolecular approach to learning disabilities.

  Bibliography: p.
  1. Learning disabilities—nutritional aspects.
2. Orthomolecular medicine. I. Title.
RJ506.L4C67   618.9'28'588071   77-22609
ISBN 0-87879-174-4

Text: 11 point Press Roman. Display: 24 point Optima Bold.
Paper: 60 pound Arbor. Cover: 10 point CIS.

6   5   4   3   2   1   0   9   8
0   9   8   7   6   5   4   3   2

contents

introduction

Learning disabilities constitute the most prevalent and urgent medical problem afflicting children not only in the United States, but in most countries of the world. The number of children involved is staggering when we consider that five percent of the nonretarded child population is affected. Physicians must be made aware that a child suffering from learning disabilities will not "outgrow it," that his condition is not "a phase he is passing through." If adequate intervention is not made into these disabilities, the child's potential will never be realized and the effects on his life will be more devastating than those of most other childhood disorders with which he might be afflicted. The earlier the diagnosis is made, the more rewarding the child's response to orthomolecular therapy or to pharmacotherapy will be, hence the more successful the results of remedial effort. Delayed diagnosis or treatment exposes the child to improper assessment by school personnel, peers, and parents, increasing the probability of permanent psychological damage.

Recent research suggests that learning disabilities are

associated with minimal brain dysfunction. This term refers to certain learning or behavioral disabilities in children of near- or above-average intelligence, ranging from mild to severe, which are associated with deviations of function of the central nervous system. There is growing recognition that the hyperactive "problem child," the child with a learning disability, may indeed be suffering from a biochemical disorder. The characteristic sign most often observed is hyperactivity—the one symptom common to all children suffering from severe disorders of behavior, learning, and communication. Other symptoms may include perceptual-motor impairments, impulsive behavior, general coordination defects, inability to concentrate, short attention span, and disorders of speech. Many children with diagnosed minimal brain dysfunction seem normal or near-normal until they enter a classroom. Then, despite average or above-average intelligence, they will have difficulty in one or more areas of learning, the most common being difficulty in reading (dyslexia). The resulting academic and emotional difficulties easily lead to misdiagnoses of retardation or of primary psychiatric problems.

The child who cannot perform on a level with his peers is a child who will in one way or another be destroyed and never achieve his full potential. He is improperly assessed by his parents, his teachers, and his classmates. The latter ultimately destroy the fragile threads of self-esteem he manages to maintain when they label him a "retard." He is finally precipitated into an emotional disorder as he progresses through each school year under the mounting stress of the demands to perform beyond his capabilities. Early recognition of his difficulties by parents and teachers can help avoid disaster by early intervention into his problems.

symptoms

While the problem of most learning-disabled children becomes manifest when they enter a school and can be detected by a kindergarten teacher, it is generally not diagnosed until the child enters the first grade. Many children progress fairly well through the early grades, but their handicaps become overt when they are introduced to subjects in which abstract thinking is required.

Learning disabilities are not disorders like the usual childhood diseases with which all parents are familiar. The signs which characterize this condition occur in groups or clusters which may vary just as children vary in other respects. Some children may have difficulty in reading because they have difficulty distinguishing letters which look alike—such as p and q, b and d—or they may have word reversals and see the word *was* when *saw* was written. Many children will be seen frequently rubbing their eyes. Other children may have disturbances in the important visual functions so necessary to reading. Their eyes may not move smoothly over the printed line because they lack smooth eye muscle control; if focusing is not properly established, they may skip words in the line, lose their place and then be unable to comprehend what they read. Problems of this nature can often be spotted by observing a child's posture as he reads or writes, for he will often cock his head at a sharp angle, keep his book on the desk, and lower his head until it is inches away from the page. Often, the child is unable to follow successive words in reading unless he moves his finger along the page under each word.

Some children show visual-motor or perceptual-motor problems in which their hands or feet cannot process the information their eyes give them. Such children cannot perform well in sports involving the need to catch a ball, to bat, kick, or throw with some degree of accuracy. They will avoid sports and show interest in solitary activities rather than subject themselves to the ridicule of their peers. Other groups of children lack fine finger control; they are unable to color and keep within the outlines of the drawing they are coloring. Because they cannot hold a pencil in a proper pincer grip, their writing is awkward—letters written above and below the line, some very small, others gigantic by comparison. Lack of fine finger control manifests itself early in the inability to cut with play scissors. Coordination of the large muscles used in running and throwing is impaired in learning-disabled children in general, they are clumsy in their movements and lack the gracefulness seen in their well-coordinated siblings. Their attention span is short and they have difficulties with memory, especially for material presented sequentially. Abstract reasoning is impossible for them or at best is very poor and disorganized.

Many parents will miss the early presumptive signs of the child at risk for learning if that child is their first-born. Only when they have a second child do they have a basis for comparison which makes the disability overt. When their overactive infant pulls himself to his feet at six months, climbs out of the crib at eight months, and is walking at ten months parents are usually pleased and often boast of this "precocious agility." Their pride turns to dismay when these "feats" are followed by the developing tornado of hyperactivity which is so often the cardinal sign of the learning-disabled child. As the learning-disabled child grows and becomes mobile, he is into everything, rushing from one thing to another, unable to concentrate or stay at anything long enough to gain anything meaningful from the experience. His attention span is short, he is easily distractible. He touches everything and overturns almost everything he touches. He may not deliberately destroy anything, but in his uncontrollable activity he frequently breaks toys and household objects. He explores every recess of the room, fingers everything, moves anything movable. The energy he exerts in whatever he does flows from an inner source which drives him relentlessly. As he grows up, he cannot rest and be tranquil, even if he wants to, for moments of peace and silence. He frequently appears clumsy in his movements. He is a disruptive influence not only in the classroom but in his home as well. Mealtimes are a nightmare of overturned glasses, spilled food, clattering cutlery, and shouting. He is the center of emotional storms which involve him and the other members of the family. He often disrupts the relations of his family members with each other.

Bedtime, the final exhausting struggle of the day, bears no resemblance to the quiet period of being tucked into bed, listening to the bedtime story, and falling quietly to sleep as Mother tiptoes from the room. The learning-disabled child is in and out of bed, may roam around the house until the early morning hours, and falls asleep when he is overcome, not by sleep, but by utter exhaustion. Or he may fall asleep and be up in a short time to awaken his parents, repeating this pattern several times during the night so that the entire family awakens exhausted each morning.

His speech and thinking processes often reveal many defects. Just as some learning-disabled children have their greatest problems with visual perception, others cannot integrate what they hear and, therefore, cannot understand, even though they do not have a measurable hearing loss. They may hear words which merely sound alike as identical, and this inability to discriminate interferes with their comprehension of what is said in conversation or of sequential commands to carry out. If, for example, the learning-disabled child with these problems is asked to "pick up the ball and then bring the book" and he hears instead the command to "pick up the bowl," he doesn't know what he must do before he brings the book. Often the development of speech in such a child may be delayed; when he does develop speech, his pronunciation may be so immature he can't be easily understood. He is rarely aware that his speech is not like that of his peers.

causes

There is no single etiological factor for learning disabilities, nor is it likely one will be found. Dr. William Wendle (1971), director of research of the New York University Institute of Rehabilitation Medicine, states that the cause seems to be malfunctioning of one area or another of the brain. In many cases, the malfunction is caused by physical damage to the brain, although the presence of such damage is difficult or impossible to prove. Because damage is subtle, states Dr. Wendle, no electroencephalogram abnormalities are found in about 50 percent of the cases. In experiments with rhesus monkeys, development of a group of 130 subjects in which asphyxia was deliberately induced during or after birth was compared with that of uninjured controls. In the early years, the differences were obvious. The asphyxiated monkeys had extreme difficulty carrying out simple motor tasks and had noticeable sensory problems. By the fourth year of life, the monkeys seemed to have made a normal adjustment, although a lack of manual dexterity and a low level of spontaneous activity were visible signs of neurological deficit. In most cases, the EEGs were normal, but autopsies showed that brain injury induced by the asphyxia had not been repaired. There was widespread nerve cell damage in several parts of the brain.

In humans, brain damage due to trauma before, during, or after birth is now believed to be responsible for many cases. The mother's health and general nutrition before conception and during pregnancy are of the utmost importance, for subtle or gross disasters occurring during these periods or during labor and delivery can compromise the child in learning and behavior (Pasamanick *et al.*, 1956).

Learning disabilities associated with minimal brain dysfunction in children of normal or superior intelligence can readily be distinguished from cases of mental retardation or of severe emotional disturbance. For this group of children, the diagnosis of *specific learning disabilities* (SLD) has been suggested. The term *general learning disabilities* should be reserved for the mentally retarded child, or the child suffering from severe disorders of behavior and communication (childhood schizophrenia, autism).

Evidence is accumulating that learning disabilities are frequently of genetic origin. Because of the worldwide scope of the problem, the World Federation of Neurology Meeting in Dallas, Texas, considered terminology related to *reading problems of genetic origin* (1968). Case studies further reveal that frequently more than one learning-disabled child is found in a single family. Additional statistics show that serious disorders of behavior, communication, and learning occur far more frequently in adopted children than in natural children. The incidence of minimal brain dysfunction with learning disabilities, furthermore, is estimated to be four to five times more frequent in boys than in girls.

A diagnosis of minimal brain dysfunction based on a cluster of deviant behaviors which include impaired concentration, short attention span, hyperactivity, impulsivity, and aggression frequently masks a borderline psychotic condition and exposes the child to an improper approach to treatment which may not only have adverse effects but may delay early intervention and proper treatment. In the genetically predisposed child, the minimal brain dysfunction syndrome can often be the early signs of schizophrenia. In eliciting a careful detailed family history during the examination of a child with minimal brain dysfunction, I have frequently found siblings described as "slow learners" or other relatives diagnosed schizophrenic, diabetic, or alcoholic. In obtaining detailed case histories of adolescent or adult schizophrenic patients, moreover, I have found a high incidence of hyperactivity and learning disabilities reported early in life. In my experience, approximately 50 percent of delinquent children and juvenile drug abusers (including alcohol abusers) suffered from a significant degree of learning disabilities in the elementary grades.

PRENATAL INFLUENCES

In his book *Life Before Birth*, Ashley Montagu states that life begins at conception and that the happenings in the interval between conception and birth are far more important for our subsequent growth and development than we have realized. The thinking about this period of the child's life had for so many years for the majority of people been rather simplistic. It was stated with confidence that the child was safe, warm, and snug in the mother's uterus, shielded and protected from all external influences while he floated in his fluid-filled sac which, by its hydraulic effect, made him safe even from physical pressures. It was believed the placenta acted as a "barrier" against the transmission of toxic substances from the mother's bloodstream.

Not until the past decade of research has it been learned that during the prenatal period—the nine months between conception and birth—a human being is more susceptible to his environment than he ever will be again in his life. What happens to him in the prenatal period can help sustain normal development or hinder him from ever achieving his full genetic potential. The events which take place before his birth can exert a lifelong influence, for part of the child's environment consists of his mother's immediate state of health, her general physical condition, her age at the time of conception, and how fatigued she becomes each day. A pregnant woman's nutrition must be more than merely adequate, it must be the best her circumstances allow.

Montagu emphasized, "A mother's nutrition is the most important single environmental influence in the life of her unborn child and by means of the food she eats a mother can have the most profound and lasting effect on her child's development—by the simple act of improving her diet where improvement is necessary she can greatly influence the development of her child toward normal healthy growth." He cites a study of malnutrition and pregnancy from which a surprising finding emerged—none of the mothers in either group, the well fed or the poorly fed, showed any signs themselves of malnutrition or deficiency disease, yet the diet of the pregnant woman can be so seriously inadequate that her child is endangered without producing any recognizable symptoms that might give warning to her or her doctors.

This finding corroborates Roger J. Williams' (1971) report that greater concern must be shown for the quality of the internal environments in which our cells and tissues function, because these environments can vary through the full spectrum, from those which barely keep cells alive up through hundreds of gradations to levels supporting something like optimal performance. It is an obvious undeniable conclusion that an unborn child should be given the advantage of growing to term in an optimum molecular environment. Proper diet based on wholesome foods, vitamin and mineral supplements, and the elimination of "junk foods" helps create such an environment for prenatal development and growth—cigarette smoking, stimulant drugs, diuretic drugs, tranquilizers, dieting with or without the use of amphetamine-containing appetite suppressors do not provide an optimum environment.

In the author's clinical practice, detailed prenatal histories and the histories of labor and delivery reveal that some complications of pregnancy and delivery occurred in a majority of the children who show evidence of brain injury, behavior disorder, or learning disabilities.

Dr. Benjamin Pasamanick (1956) and his coworkers, in a series of papers describing their research in these areas, postulated "a continuum of reproductive casualties extending from fetal deaths through a descending gradient of brain damage manifested in cerebral palsy, epilepsy, mental deficiency and behavior disorders in childhood." Dr. Pasamanick (1958) extended the continuum of reproductive casualties to include reading disorders in childhood. They compared the prenatal and birth records of 372 white male children with reading disorders born in Baltimore between 1935 and 1945 with the records of a similar number of matched controls. The results of the study "appear to indicate there exists a relationship between certain abnormal conditions associated with birth and the subsequent development of reading disorders in the child."

Those children with reading disorders had a significantly larger proportion of premature births and abnormalities of the prenatal and delivery periods than their control subjects. They found the toxemias of pregnancy and bleeding during pregnancy constituted those complications largely responsible for the differences between the two groups. The investigation suggested some of the learning disabilities in children constitute a component in the continuum of reproductive casualties, which Pasamanick had previously hypothesized to be composed of a lethal component consisting of stillbirths and neonatal deaths and a sublethal component consisting of cerebral palsy, epilepsy, mental deficiency, and behavior disorders in children.

Impressions leading to similar conclusions were formed from the author's clinical experiences based on detailed histories of hundreds of learning-disabled children. The interview with the parents generally begins with the request that they describe the pregnancy. With very few exceptions in the hundreds of pairs of parents interviewed, the opening response is "the pregnancy was perfectly normal." It is appalling to contemplate the disasters which can await the child in what women have been led to believe are quite the usual and, therefore, normal experiences of pregnancy. Many mothers report with a feeling of pride their accomplishment of having carried a pregnancy to full term and delivered a baby of normal weight without having gained a single pound in nine months of the pregnancy! Nausea and vomiting occurs in the great majority of mothers and is accepted as a normal occurrence. Many mothers attempt to minimize the importance of "morning sickness" by adding, "but I was sick every day with all my pregnancies."

Many mothers reported dieting severely thoughout the pregnancy at the demand of their doctor, because he preferred his patients have small babies. Amphetamines were frequently prescribed to suppress the appetite or to combat fatigue. Tranquilizer and sedative medications were used freely throughout the pregnancies, but the most frequently prescribed medication seemed to be the diuretic drugs which mothers took throughout the pregnancies and which were in very few cases taken along with an increase in potassium-rich foods. Anemia during pregnancy was frequently reported.

The frequency of occurrence of complications during the perinatal period is higher in children with learning disabilities. A prolonged period of labor and a difficult delivery is the most commonly encountered history in the birth record of a learning-disabled child. In a study reported by Dr. Mary Hoffman (1971), 25 percent of a group of children who were failing students were products of difficult deliveries, while this occurred in only 1.5 percent of the histories of the able students. Cyanosis occurred in 11 percent of the learning disabled and in only 0.5 percent of the able students. Prolonged labor, blood incompatibility, premature births, postmature births, breech deliveries, and induced labor were also found to be highly significant factors in the historical background of children with learning disabilities, since these casualties occurred far more frequently than in able children.

Even though research cannot at this time give an unequivocal or full answer to the question of what effect malnutrition or malnourishment has on intellectual development, this is not a valid reason to delay programs for improving the nutritional status and eating practices of mothers and infants. Information demonstrating the benefits of good nutrition in improved health, physical growth, and improved learning already justify such efforts.

VISUAL FUNCTIONS

The examination of a child who suffers from a disorder of speech, communication, or learning cannot be considered complete without a visual examination, for the investigation of sight and vision is as important as any other part of the total examination and more important and revealing than many other routines. A major number of the children treated by the author have all had examinations which included electroencephalograms, but very few have been examined for vision by a vision specialist. If an examination had been done, it was performed for sight, and if the child demonstrated 20/20 vision on the Snellen Chart, the parents were informed there was nothing wrong with the child's eyes. This may be true for distance eyesight, but overlooks all the near-point visual activity so important to the dynamic visual process of reading (Wunderlich 1970). The child who has a school or learning problem must have an examination performed by a specialist who investigates the function of the eyes as well

17

as their structure. Such a specialist could be an opthalmologist (an M.D. specializing in diseases of the eye) or an optometrist specializing in developmental vision. At the present time, few ophthalmologists perform these examinations, so one is more apt to find a developmental vision specialist among optometrists. Sight is the ability of the eye to see clearly. It refers only to the ability to resolve detail. Vision is the ability to gain meaning from what is seen (Wunderlich 1970).

Too often parents are lulled into a false sense of security when they are told that their child's eyes are "fine," for here, also, early detection and treatment will produce a more rewarding response and the results of the remedial efforts will be more successful. As just mentioned, there can be significant deviations from normal vision even if a child has 20/20 on the Snellen Chart. Farsightedness can be overlooked in a distance vision screening examination, for example, and can cause difficulties when a child does near work. There can be problems if one eye is different from the other in refractive power. Convergence of the eyes noseward for looking at things close up is also of vital importance in centering with two eyes on a near-point task. Convergence bears an important relationship to focusing: the two processes are combined. If this link is not proper, a child can be out of focus and be completely unaware that he is, just as a child who sees a separate image with each eye has no way of telling us about this since he believes everyone sees in this way. The out-of-focus child cannot tell us about his blurred vision until he can be helped to see in sharp focus with the aid of lenses.

The author has seen many children who had not seen near things in sharp focus or looked at the world through binocular vision until their eyes had been treated successfully by a developmental optometrist or by an ophthalmologist interested in developmental vision. Yet these children are daily trying to learn to read when the printed page presents nothing but a blur. Lack of smooth eye muscle control makes a difficult task of trying to follow successive words in a line of print as the eyes sweep across a page. Often the eyes will not make the repeated necessary convergences if the focusing is not proper; and the child will skip words in the line, lose his place, or be unable to find the first word on the next line and as a result will not comprehend what he reads. Significantly, hyperactivity is frequently reduced when the visual systems work efficiently.

Developmental visual training is another vital link in the creation of an optimum molecular environment for the mind. Neither improved nutrition, vitamin and mineral supplements, enriched educational opportunities, or visual and perceptual motor training alone can be successful in fully helping the child with learning disabilities. All must be used in a coordinated program to develop each child's potential.

treatment

Even with early intervention, many of the effects of learning disabilities cannot be overcome with the best help now available. While much emphasis has been placed on the neurogenic learning disorders, however, other important variables in the learning process have been overlooked or ignored (Cott 1972).

The author would like to present for consideration a most important variable—the biochemical disorders which interfere with learning—and a new adjunct to treatment which involves the use of large doses of vitamins, minerals, and the maintenance of proper nutrition to create the optimum molecular environment for the brain. Drugs are being used widely as the primary intervention for the treatment of learning disabilities and are of importance in helping many children.

In January, 1971 the Office of Child Development and the Office of the Assistant Secretary for Health and Scientific Affairs, Department of Health Education and Welfare, called a conference to discuss the use of stimulant medications in the treatment of elementary school-age children with certain behavioral disturbances. Public concern was increasing about the increasing use of stimulant medications in treating so-called hyperkinetic behavior disorders. Questions were raised by concerned parents whether these drugs, which were widely abused by adolescents and adults, were truly safe for children. Were they properly prescribed, or were they used for children who in fact need other types of treatment? Was emphasis on prescribing medications to alleviate behavior disorders misleading?

To clarify the conditions in which these medications were beneficial or harmful to children, HEW's Office of Child Development invited a panel of fifteen specialists drawn from relevant fields to meet in Washington D.C. to review the evidence of research and experience and prepare an advisory report for professionals and the public. Their report dealt with the wide range of conditions and disabilities which can interfere with a child's learning and highlighted such etiologic factors as social deprivations, stress at home or at school, mental retardation, childhood psychosis, and autism. Other factors included were medical conditions such as blindness, deafness, or obvious brain dysfunction. Some cases were described as associated with specific reading or perceptual defects and others with severe personality or emotional disturbance.

They clearly defined hyperactivity as physical activity which appears driven as if there were an "inner tornado." Thus, the activity is beyond the child's control, as compared to other children. The child is distracted, racing from one idea and interest to another, unable to focus attention.

They continued that the fact that these dysfunctions range from mild to severe and have ill-understood causes and outcomes should *not* obscure the necessity for skilled and special interventions. Attention was drawn to the similarity in the majority of better known diseases—from cancer and diabetes to hypertension—which have multiple or unknown causes and consequences. Their early manifestations are often not readily recognizable, yet useful treatment programs have been developed to alleviate these conditions. Uncertainty as to cause has not prevented tests of the effectiveness of available treatments while the search for clearer definitions and more effective kinds of therapy continues. The panel suggested the same principles should clearly apply to the hyperkinetic behavior disorders.

The focus of the HEW panel's report was on issues related to the use of drugs in treating learning disabilities. They concluded that stimulant medications are beneficial in only about one half to two thirds of the cases in which use of the drugs is warranted. They considered the stimulant drugs to be the first and least complicated of the medicines to be tried, while other medications—the so-called tranquilizers and antidepressants—should be generally reserved for a smaller group of patients. They agreed the medications did not "cure" the condition, but the child may become more accessible to educational and counseling efforts. Over the short term and at a critical age, this can provide the help needed for the child's development.

The panel emphasized the rights of parents and took the position that under no circumstances should any attempt be made to coerce the parents to accept any particular treatment and that the consent of the patient and his parents or guardian must be obtained for treatment. They further added that it is proper for school personnel to inform parents of a child's behavioral problems, but members of the school staff should not directly diagnose hyperkinetic disturbance or prescribe treatment. The school should initiate contact with a physician only with the parent's consent. The report was concluded with the summary that there is a place for stimulant medications in the treatment of the hyperkinetic behavioral disturbance, but these medications are *not* the only form of effective treatment.

The author agrees in essence with the conference report. Early intervention is of the utmost importance if the hyperkinetic learning-disabled child is to have an opportunity to learn and achieve. It is true in most instances the hyperactivity will subside spontaneously by age twelve or thirteen, but those parents who accepted the advice their child would "outgrow" the condition find it is too late for him. His academic career is gone, and opportunities for work later in life are indeed limited, since there are very few jobs left which do not require a degree of literacy.

It is unfortunate that the H E W panel, while pointing out that drugs were not the only effective treatment, was not convened to report on effective alternatives to drug treatment or effective treatments for that one third to one half of five million children who are not helped by drugs.

There is rapidly accumulating evidence that a child's ability to learn can be improved by the use of large doses of certain vitamins, mineral supplements, and by improvement of his general nutritional status through removal of "junk foods" and additives from his daily diet.

Orthomolecular treatment has been described by Dr. Linus Pauling, in his classical paper on orthomolecular psychiatry (1968), as treatment of illness by the provision of the optimum molecular composition of the brain, especially the optimum concentration of substances normally present in the human body. The implications for much-needed research in the more universal application of orthomolecular treatment are clear.

In the author's experience, orthomolecular intervention with the hyperkinetic learning-disabled child can help better than 50 percent. These statistics achieve greater significance when it is considered that the children treated have failed to improve with the use of Ritalin or amphetamines. In such cases, many parents were searching for an alternative to drug therapy because their children were experiencing the side effects of insomnia, loss of appetite with concomitant weight loss, reduction in rate of growth, a reaction of fatigue and sedation, or irritability and tearfulness when the dr was given in doses large enough to control the hyperactivity.

Many children had been put on a regime of various psychotropic (tranquilizer) medications which failed because they produced the paradoxical effect of overstimulation and increased the hyperactivity and disturbed behavior.

Many parents who had read of the orthomolecular approach or had spoken to other parents whose children were achieving notable improvement on the regime sought this as the primary treatment. Since the orthomolecular approach is compatible with all other substances used in the drug intervention, and since the megavitamins potentiate the action of most drugs, the treatments can be combined. This is frequently done early in treatment, while the vitamin doses are gradually being raised to the optimal maintenance level and more rapid control of the hyperactivity is required. At times, tranquilizer medication is added at the request or insistence of the school authorities to bring the hyperactive, disruptive behavior under more rapid control.

The large majority of children treated by the orthomolecular approach improve without the use of drugs. Fortunately, very few parents accept the cliches with which their concerns about their child's development are met by so many of their pediatricians and family physicians. They are not satisfied with such palliatives as "boys are slower than girls," "you're an anxious mother, your baby is fine," "lots of healthy children do not speak until they are four years old," or "there's nothing to worry about if your baby creeps backward or rolls from place to place." In the author's experience, the mothers most often were first to notice their child's problems; only in a very low percentage of cases was their pediatrician first to make the diagnosis. Many parents, after reading about the orthomolecular approach, instituted the recommended dietary changes and found that these changes alone brought about a dramatic reduction in hyperactivity. Other parents purchased vitamins and reported improvement when their child was given several of the vitamins used in the treatment.

During the treatment of many hundreds of psychotic children, the author noted and reported that in most cases in which parents persisted in the proper administration of the vitamins and the diet, significant improvement in many areas of functioning was achieved. The most significant and earliest sign of improvement reported by the parents was a decrease in hyperactivity, which led to improved concentration and attention span with a resultant improved capacity for learning. Trials with the orthomolecular treatment were then begun in children exhibiting specific learning disabilities, the child diagnosed hyperkinetic or minimal brain dysfunction.

With orthomolecular treatment, results are frequently quick and the reduction in hyperactivity often dramatic, but in most instances several months elapse before significant changes are seen. The child exhibits, among other qualities, a willingness to cooperate with his parents and teachers. These changes are seen in the majority of children who failed to improve with the use of the stimulant drugs or tranquilizer medications. The majority of the children the author sees have been exposed to every form of treatment and every known tranquilizer and sedative, with little or no success even in controlling the hyperactivity. Concentration and attention span increases, and the child is able to work productively for increasingly longer periods of time. He ceases to be an irritant to his teacher and classmates. Early intervention is of the utmost importance, not only for the child, but for the entire family, since the child suffering from minimal brain dysfunction is such a devastating influence on the family constellation. He is the matrix of emotional storms which envelop every member of the household and disrupt both their relationship to him and to each other.

Until orthomolecular studies were begun, most remedial specialists stressed the more peripheral aspects of a handicapped child's performance and ignored the biochemical basis of his disturbed behavior and impaired ability to learn. In this means of intervention, remedial efforts are directed toward both brain function and body chemistry. In addition to the employment of perceptual motor techniques and pharmacotherapy, attempts should be made to improve the child's biochemical balance through the use of orthomolecular techniques (Cott 1971). Improvement under the orthomolecular treatment is directing the attention of the scientific community to the central processes and closer scrutiny of the biochemical processes of the learning-disabled child.

MEGAVITAMINS

Based on empirical data, the application of orthomolecular principles can be successful in helping many learning-disabled children. Positive results have been obtained when the treatment regimen consisted of the following vitamins: niacinamide (vitamin B-3) or niacin (vitamin B-3), 1 to 2 grams daily, depending on body weight; vitamin C, 1 to 2 grams daily; pyridoxine (vitamin B-6), 200 to 300 mg. daily; calcium pantothenate, 200 to 400 mg. daily; B-complex 50, half a tablet. The vitamins are generally administered twice daily. Magnesium is frequently used for its calming effect on hyperactivity, and to prevent a depletion of this important mineral by the large doses of pyridoxine.

These are starting doses for children weighing 35 pounds or more. If a child weighs less than 35 pounds, 1 gram daily of niacinamide and vitamin C are used in half-gram doses administered twice daily. If the child shows no signs of intolerance after two weeks, the dose is increased to twice the amount. For a child weighing 45 pounds or more, an optimum daily maintenance level of about 3 grams of niacinamide and 3 grams of vitamin C is reached. Frequently, vitamin B-12, vitamin E, riboflavin (B-2), thiamine (B-1), folic acid, and B-15 can be valuable additions to the treatment. No serious side effects have resulted in any of the thousands of children treated with these substances. The side effects which occur infrequently are dose related and subside with the reduction of the dose.

SIDE EFFECTS: NIACIN AND NIACINAMIDE

Niacin can elevate blood glucose levels and levels of uric acid. These side effects are very infrequent and the parameters return to normal with a reduction of the dose or with discontinuation of the niacin and the substitution of niacinamide. For two or three days after beginning its use, niacin will produce a feeling of warmth in the body, a flushing of the skin comparable to a mild sunburn, sometimes accompanied by itching. These symptoms occur fifteen to twenty minutes after taking the medication and subside in one to two hours; they recur with each succeeding dose, but with diminished intensity. This effect no longer appears after the second or third day of administration of niacin.

Niacinamide, the preferred form of vitamin B-3 for use in children, does not produce these symptoms. Headaches of the temporal variety, however, may occur and will respond to reduction of the dose. Both niacin and niacinamide may produce nausea. While this side effect occurs very infrequently, it is the most common side effect and, like other side effects of the megavitamins, responds to a reduction in dose. In the treatment of 8,000 adults, swelling of the face or ankles occurred in six patients and a brownish patchy discoloration of the skin occurred in five, but neither of these side effects occurred in the treatment of 2,000 children. The side effects cleared when niacinamide was substituted for niacin.

SIDE EFFECTS: VITAMIN C

The major side effects of vitamin C are increased frequency of urination and mild diarrhea. These occur infrequently and respond to reduction of the dose. Some children can be intolerant of vitamin C and are treated instead with sodium ascorbate, which does not produce side effects.

SIDE EFFECTS: PYRIDOXINE

Dr. Paul Gyorgy, who discovered B-6, indicates that it is quite safe even at high dosage levels. In 1966, the American Academy of Pediatrics reviewed the use of B-6 and concluded that "to date there had been no report of deleterious effects associated with ingestion of large doses of vitamin B-6 (0.2-1 gram daily)."

SIDE EFFECTS: CALCIUM PANTOTHENATE

This vitamin is reported by Dr. Roger Williams, its discoverer, to be non toxic even in multiple gram doses. He reported monkeys to have ingested five hundred times their normal intake of this vitamin with no adverse effects. He reports the life-span of mice given supplements of calcium pantothenate daily to have averaged 645 days as compared with 549 days for mice treated alike but given only a good commercial laboratory mouse diet.

AVAILABILITY:

The vitamins are available as tablets, capsules, or liquids. Often side effects may be produced by the fillers which are used in making tablets. Fillers are most often sugar, corn-starch, and a variety of chemical substances all of which can produce side effects. Tablets are available without these fillers, however. Capsules are less likely to contain fillers, since pure vitamin powders can be used in the manufacture of capsules. Liquid vitamins are the least preferred form to use, since all liquid medicinal preparations must contain preservatives, mold retardants, and glycerine, which is used to prevent freezing in shipment. Even more harmful for the hyperactive child are the artificial colors, artificial flavors, and sweeteners used in the preparation of liquid medications. If a child cannot swallow tablets or capsules, the tablets may be crushed and stirred into juice or some other food which would make the mixture palatable. None of the children treated have ever developed a serious side effect from mega-vitamins.

It has been shown that proper brain function requires adequate tissue respiration, and Dr. O. Warburg (1966), Nobel laureate in biochemistry, described the importance of vitamins B-3 and C in the respiration of all body tissues in the maintenance of health and proper function.

Laboratory findings with animals have shown a direct relationship between vitamin intake and learning enhancement. It has been found by some researchers that injections of vitamin B-12 markedly enhanced learning in rats.

IMPORTANCE OF DIETARY CONTROL

Control of diet is an integral part of the total treatment of a learning-disabled child and failure to improve the nutritional status can be responsible for achieving minimal results. Greater concern must be shown for the quality of the child's internal environment in which his cells and tissues function if we are to help him attain optimal performance. The removal of offending foods from the diet of disturbed or learning-disabled children can result in dramatic improvement in behavior, attention span, and concentration.

The role of diets deficient in essential nutrients has been well documented as the cause of vitamin deficiency diseases such as beriberi and scurvy. The former is the result of a deficiency of thiamine (vitamin B-1); the latter a deficiency of vitamin C. The role of improper diet as a causative factor in the production of disturbed behavior became clear when the discovery was made that pellagra was produced by a diet deficient in niacin. In the late stages of the illness, which begins with a widespread skin eruption, the patient develops symptoms resembling those of schizophrenia, including perceptual distortions and a disorder in thinking and behavior. When niacin was added to the patient's diet, pellagra receded completely.

Children or adults suffering from hypoglycemia must eat a diet richest in protein foods, moderate fat, and low in carbohydrate foods. Cane sugar and those carbohydrate foods quickly converted to glucose must be eliminated, for they exert a definite influence on brain chemistry and overstimulate the pancreas to overproduce insulin. A study at M.I.T. (March 1975) revealed the relationship in brain tissue in rats between the amounts of neurotransmitters present in the brain and the presence or absence of protein in each meal. The daily increases or decreases in the dietary intake of certain amino acids found in foods affect the production of neurotransmitters which stimulate impulses from one brain cell to the next. It was also reported that insulin apparently sequesters some amino acids.

Cane sugar and foods prepared with sugar are offending foods for all children, normal as well as disabled. The physical manifestations of conditions produced by including cane sugar in the child's diet are well documented and known to many parents. Dentists report children with a high intake of cane sugar have more cavities. Sugar-loaded foods spoil a child's appetite for good, nutritious foods and keep him literally "addicted" to sugar in all forms: cookies, cakes, ice cream, soda pop, and the great multitude of sugar-frosted cereals which become the basic foods in his unbalanced diet. Overlooked, however, have been the equally devastating effects which such a sugar-loaded diet has on a child's *behavior*. In the treatment of children suffering from disorders of behavior or learning disabilities, I have found a significant percentage were dramatically improved by removing sugar and other junk foods from their diet. Those parents who were successful in enforcing the cane sugar-free diet achieved great success in helping their children overcome the hyperactive behavior that was interfering with learning and peer relationships. Most of the sweetened foods also contain artificial colors and artificial flavors, to which many children react with an allergy not manifested in the usual ways but by sudden outbursts of disturbed, disruptive behavior produced by a reaction in the brain. A high percentage of children have some disturbance of glucose metabolism; in this group, the eating of sugar-laden foods produces an initial rise in blood sugar level which is normal, but this rise is followed in an hour or two by a precipitous drop in blood sugar level to a point lower than the level at the time the sugar was eaten. This drop interferes with the levels of transmitters which control sleep, mood, motivation, and learning, and results in overactive and, at times, violent disruptive behavior (Yaryura-Tobias *et al.* 1975). When a child has been following a sugar-free diet for a period of time and his behavior has improved, members of his family know when he has had sweets by the return of his previous irritability and overactivity. I have seen a number of children who reacted to the withdrawal of sugar from their diet with the personality change and physical discomfort seen during withdrawal of drugs. Wheat products and milk, which so frequently occur in foods containing sugar, are highly allergenic for many children and often produce cerebral allergies which are manifested by disturbed behavior.

Since many disturbed and learning-disabled children are found to have either hypoglycemia, hyperinsulinism, or dysinsulinism, cane sugar and rapidly absorbed carbohydrate foods should be eliminated from their diets. It has been the universal observation of those investigators who assess the nutritional status of such children that they eat a diet which is richest in sugar, candy, sweets, and foods made with sugar. The removal of these foods results in a dramatic decrease in hyperactivity. Most children do not drink milk unless it is sweetened with chocolate syrup or some other syrupy additive. All the beverages they consume every day are spiked with sugar: soda, caffeinated cola drinks, highly sweetened "fruit juice," and other concoctions which are sold to them by television commercials. The child who drinks any water at all is indeed rare.

The appalling fact about the constant consumption of these "junk foods" is the parents' belief that these foods are good for their children. Parents must realize that they litter their children's bodies by making unnatural foods available to them and incorporating them in their daily diet. Because children will not voluntarily exclude such foods from their diet, they must be helped to accomplish this; these foods should not be brought into the home. The child must learn the principles of proper nutrition and proper eating from his parents. The dissemination of this knowledge is far too important to entrust it to the writers of television commercials whose aim is to sell, not educate.

Dr. Jean Mayer, Professor of Nutrition at Harvard University, speaking at a 1970 symposium on hunger and malnutrition, stated that "studies at Harvard among resident physicians suggest that the average physician knows little more about nutrition than the average secretary, unless the secretary has a weight problem, and then she probably knows more than the average physician. We did find that there is a difference between older and younger physicians in relation to this problem. The older doctors do not know more about nutrition than their younger colleagues, but they are conscious of this lack. All in all, it seems that most physicians tend to be happy about this state of affairs." Dr. Mayer complained that "only a half dozen or so medical schools in the United States include a nutrition course in the curriculum. Nutrition education should be centered on foods—their size, shape, color, caloric value, etc.—we must relate such vital information to the everyday uses of all people."

The author has taken many dietary histories which revealed the usual "nutritious" breakfast for some children consists of a glass of soda or "coke" and a portion of choco-late layer cake! For the child with hypoglycemia, such food assures a drop in blood glucose level for several hours, during which time the child's brain function is impaired so he can-not learn well even if he does not suffer from learning dis-abilities. At best, the breakfast menu of the majority of learning-disabled children is poorly balanced and varies from the just-mentioned extreme by the substitution of sugar-frosted cereals. Glucose in the bloodstream is one of the most important nutrients for proper brain function, and the main-tenance of a proper glucose level is essential in the creation of an optimum molecular environment for the mind.

An increasingly greater awareness of the importance of the role of nutrition in health maintenance led to more re-search which revealed that, beyond malnutrition due to lack of food or proper diet, there were illnesses or conditions pro-duced by perfectly good foods which are offending foods for the brain chemistry of many children and adults, capable of producing mental or physical symptoms. These foods may be the basic staples in the daily well-balanced diet of a hyper-active child, yet they produce disturbed, hyperactive be-havior, or physical symptoms.

Many wholesome foods can be offensive for minimal-brain-dysfunction children. Their response is an allergic one, but the symptoms produced by the allergy are not the usual allergic symptoms but a *disturbance in behavior.* This re-sponse must be considered the result of a cerebral allergy. The foods most often productive of cerebral allergies are wheat, milk, eggs, corn and corn products (the latter are al-most as ubiquitous as sugar), and beef. Since these foods are consumed daily and many are used several times each day, we can see dramatic changes in behavior when the offending food or foods are removed from the diet. The reduction in hyperactivity can in many cases be immediate. This can be accomplished by an elimination diet and I have found the foods most often responsible are those which the child eats or drinks most often and in the largest amounts. I have found few instances in which a half-gallon-a-day milk drinker was not benefited by being withdrawn completely from milk. Other liquids consumed in prodigious amounts are apple juice and soda. I have seen many children whose daily allotment of 48 ounces of soda was consumed by noon each day. These are the sodas of which Jean Mayer said that the labels listing the chemical additives, artificial colors, flavors, and preservatives read like a qualitative analysis of a water sample drawn from New York's East River.

Dr. Curtis Dohan, Professor of Medicine at the University of Pennsylvania, conducted studies with disturbed adult schizophrenic patients hospitalized in the Veterans Administration hospital in Coatesville, Pennsylvania, and reported that a cereal-free and milk-free diet added to the daily treatment regime improved those patients more rapidly than those who were continued on the usual institutional fare which included cereal grains and milk. Dr. Dohan's original study, which drew criticism, was replicated in a recent study (1976). Schizophrenics maintained on a cereal-free and milk-free diet and receiving optimal treatment with neuroleptics showed an interruption or reversal of their therapeutic progress during a period of "blind" wheat gluten challenge. The exacerbation of the disease process was not due to variations in the drug doses. After termination of the wheat gluten challenge, the course of improvement was reinstated. The observed effects seemed to be due to a primary schizophrenia-promoting effect of wheat gluten.

Dr. Ben Feingold's work with salicylate-sensitive children and their response to the removal of artificial colors, flavors, and foods with naturally occurring salicylates is well known. This subgroup of minimal-brain-dysfunction children responds dramatically to the elimination of these additives which occur in sodas, most frankfurters, and other luncheon meats, as well as in wholesome foods such as apples, oranges, peaches, grapes, raisins, cucumbers, pickles, and many others.

Orthomolecular treatment has many advantages which make it especially suitable for large numbers of children. Treatment can be directed by parents and paraprofessionals, reducing to a minimum the occasions upon which the child must be brought to a specialist for therapy. It is inexpensive, as it does not depend upon complex machinery or equipment, or upon the long-term use of psychotropic drugs. Of great importance is the role orthomolecular treatment could serve as a preventive as well as a therapeutic measure, because it could easily be included in prenatal and infant care programs everywhere. These are important considerations in view of the evidence that neurologically based and biochemically based learning disabilities are especially frequent among children from low-income areas. Bronfenbrenner (1969) points out that a low-income mother's "exposure to nutritional deficiency, illness, fatigue, or emotional stress can be far more damaging to her child than was previously thought. The neurological disturbances thus produced persist through early childhood into the school years, where they are reflected in impaired learning capacity."

The relationship of severe infant malnutrition to infant mortality, disease, and retardation in physical development are all well documented. In recent years evidence has accumulated that malnutrition has adverse effects on mental development and learning as well. Mild malnutrition can result in a child who is a "picky eater" who chronically gags when he swallows some food, or swallows it readily and then vomits. Recent studies utilized such reported differences within young twin pairs to show that subtle variations in eating habits in the first year can be related to differences in mental abilities later in life.

TRACE MINERALS

The fact that chemical substances can affect behavior

has been apparent since the discovery of alcoholic fermentation and, in recent times, has been emphasized by the therapeutic use and nonmedical abuse of psychotropic and hallucinogenic drugs such as LSD. Abnormal behavior can result from dietary deficiencies of such trace minerals as copper, calcium, magnesium, manganese, and zinc. Dr. Carl Pfeiffer, Director of the Brain Bio-Center in Princeton, New Jersey, has reported clinical improvement in a subgroup of the schizophrenic population when he reestablished proper balances of copper and zinc by administering supplements of these minerals. Zinc deficiency in pregnant rats produced loss of appetite and, in the fetus, decreased levels of DNA in the brain, decreased total body and liver zinc levels, and caused retardation in growth. Cobalt, zinc, and manganese serve as cofactors for various metabolic enzymes; iron is an integral component of hemoglobin. Magnesium activates approximately 100 enzyme chains in every cell in the body. Zinc activates 60 of these chains; copper, 12; cobalt, 16; manganese, 20; iron, 30.

At the annual meeting of the American Psychiatric Association in 1976, Dr. David C. Jimerson reported that spinal fluid calcium levels are significantly correlated with symptom severity in depressed patients, although mean calcium levels did not differ from control groups. Calcium levels showed a significant negative correlation with the accumulations of the dopamine metabolite homovanillic acid, suggesting a relationship between depressed calcium levels and the function of brain transmitters. Excess of copper in the tissues can lead to zinc and pyridoxine deficiencies (Pfeiffer 1974). The resulting zinc deficiency may lead to an accumulation of vitamin A in the liver and a shortage of vitamin A in blood plasma. Deficiency of pyridoxine leads to a shortage of B-3, which in turn produces a deficiency of nicotinamide adenodinucleotide, which is converted to tryptophan. There has been insufficient clinical application of research findings of the effects of trace minerals, in spite of increasing evidence that an analysis of trace metal concentrations can be diagnostically significant. Ross Seasly of the Kettering Medical Center, for example, notes that during the last ten years Kettering's clinical laboratory has never received a request for an analysis of trace metal concentrations.

Magnesium, like calcium, is a metal of considerable physiologic importance; in the mammalian organism, it is indispensable to life. Magnesium affects the activity of numerous enzyme systems; it is slowly absorbed from the gastrointestinal tract and rapidly excreted by the kidney. Therefore, ingestion of foods containing magnesium have no particular influence on the blood magnesium level. Clinically, low levels of magnesium in the blood plasma are associated with states of hyperexcitability, while high levels of magnesium have a sedative and depressant effect. Serum magnesium levels have considerable normal fluctuation and persistently low or high magnesium values may be present without any clinical abnormality.

TOXIC METALS

Brain catecholamines, or neurotransmitters, regulate mood and behavior and influence aggressiveness and stereotyped repetitive behavior.

The environmental pollutants are often heavy metals such as lead, mercury, or cadmium. The lead pollution of our environment, and particularly our cities, has already reached a disturbingly high level. In 1967 in Manchester, England, a group of children were found to have lead levels of 30+ micrograms per 100 mg. of blood. Professor D. Bryce-Smith of the University of Reading recently wrote (1974) that no other chemical pollutant has accumulated in man to average levels so close to the threshold for overt clinical poisoning. Whenever lead poisoning has been diagnosed, it has always been traced to some definite source; in children it may be chewing on old paint work or toys containing lead. There has been no known case of lead poisoning, however, from the widespread general pollution to which everyone is exposed. This is why the apparently alarming situation to which Professor Bryce-Smith draws attention has caused little concern. Lead pollution does not seem to be doing any serious damage, the complacent argument runs, so why worry about it? This position, however, begins to look increasingly vulnerable in the face of mounting evidence that lead could have harmful effects at levels well below those which cause overt poisoning.

In 1964, Sir Alan Moncrieff and others at the Institute of Child Health in London found a group of mentally retarded children had distinctly more lead in their blood than a group of normal children. In fact, nearly half of the retarded children had higher blood levels than the maximum level in the other group. It does not, of course, follow that lead was responsible for the children's mental retardation. It could well have been their retardation which made them more prone to chew on substances with a lead content. Nevertheless, the possibility that lead at levels too low to cause obvious poisoning could result in mental retardation was one that could not be ignored. The findings acted as a spur to the search for some measurable effect of low levels of lead in the human body.

In 1970, Dr. Sven Hernberg and his associates found lead affected the functioning of an enzyme, ALA dehydratase, which is involved in haem (the precursor of hemoglobin) synthesis. Furthermore, he showed that in the test tube any level of lead affected the activity of ALA dehydratase to some degree. In October, 1970, a research group lead by J. A. Millar fed lead to baby rats and found the activity of ALA dehydratase was affected not only in their blood, but in their brains as well. They wrote in their report in the *Lancet*, "The finding of decreased ALA dehydratase activity in the blood of children with lead levels falling within the normal range, and the possibility that similar biochemical changes are present in the brain also, emphasizes the danger of exposure to even very small amounts of lead during childhood and suggests that a downward revision of acceptable levels of blood lead in children is desirable." In addition to lead discharged into the atmosphere in vehicle exhaust, people also absorb lead from foods, water, and many other sources.

It is now a well-known clinical fact that susceptibility to the harmful effects of lead is highly variable. Lead in heavy concentrations in the tissues (and some of the hundreds of children I have examined have concentrations as high as 85 parts per million) can interfere with metabolic reactions which activate other metals such as copper, iron, manganese, and potassium.

In studies of the toxic metals in children's hair, the author found that children show a higher concentration of lead than do adults. In adult groups, it has been reported pregnant women show a greater susceptibility than other adult members of the population. Now that attention has been focused on the level of lead in the tissues of many middle-class Americans who may be exposed to lead byproducts in gasoline exhaust fumes, many new cases of borderline lead toxicity are appearing without the usual explanation of lead ingestion. While a close correlation exists between the level of atmospheric lead and the levels of lead accumulated and stored in the body, there is a wide diversity in the susceptibility, not only to symptoms, but also to accumulation of this toxic trace metal. Recent experiments again give evidence that nutritional factors, particularly dietary calcium, may be important determinants in the capacity of the body to absorb and retain lead. Animals receiving lead in their drinking water showed a greater absorption of lead when their diet was deficient in calcium. This group of animals absorbed four times as much lead compared to the group which received a normal dietary calcium intake Lead is everywhere in our environment. Each year the average car spews out about two kilograms of lead from its exhaust. While lead is not highly toxic like cadmium, its presence in such large amounts adds to the dangers it presents. The automobile is not alone responsible for enveloping the earth in an envelope of lead. Ice borings at the polar ice cap revealed that samples of ice layers deposited decades before the advent of the internal combustion engine and leaded gasoline contained lead.

Children breathe lead and accumulate it from sucking their dirty fingers and toys, from inhaling road dust and airplane exhaust, and from many other sources. Children can absorb dangerous quantities of lead from chewing newspaper or color-printed pages in magazines. At present one quarter of several hundred thousand children tested and living in cities have blood levels at the borderline of toxicity.

Dr. Caprio and his associates (1974) studied the blood levels of 5226 children living near the congested traffic lanes of Newark and reported those children living closest to the highways had the highest levels of lead in their blood. Some had poisonous levels of lead.

While the chronic ingestion of lead has yet to be clearly associated with hyperactivity, two recently reported studies of mice and rats showed that lead produces definite changes in brain chemistry. Such changes may lead to behavioral disorders including hyperactivity (Michaelson 1973).

At the University of Cincinnati Medical Center, Drs. I. R. Michaelson and Mitchell U. Sauerhoff administered varying concentrations of lead solution to nursing mother rats and then measured neurochemical changes in 90 babies. They found 15 to 20 percent decreases in brain dopamine. At Johns Hopkins University, Drs. Ellen K. Silbergeld and Alan M. Goldberg (1973) tested the effects of lead ingestion on mouse behavior; after administering lead solutions to nursing mothers, the investigators found the offspring were retarded in development and suffered behavior disorders. They were hyperactive and aggressive. The animals did not, however, exhibit signs of lead poisoning. It was reported the behavioral effects were due to abnormalities in the concentration of serotonin in the brain and with alterations in the metabolism of norepinephrine.

In a study reported in the *American Journal of Psychiatry* (David *et al.* 1976), lead-chelating medication was used to treat 13 hyperkinetic school children whose blood and urine lead levels were in an elevated but "nontoxic" range. Six children with histories of etiologically relevant perinatal or developmental complications showed relatively little improvement. Seven other children with unremarkable histories, and for whom a lead etiology could thus be entertained, showed marked improvement. The authors conclude that lead may play an important role in the etiology of some cases of hyperactivity; and the medical workup of hyperactivity should include lead level measurements and careful consideration of other possible etiological factors.

Of equally great importance as a pollutant and more lethal than lead is cadmium. High ratios of cadmium to zinc in the kidney have been associated with death from hypertension. Injection of a zinc chelate into cadmium hypertensive rats resulted in a return of the hypertension to normal levels. Vitamin C is effective against cadmium-produced anemia.

Recent research showed zinc and selenium to be protective against the accumulation of lethal doses of cadmium. The accumulation of toxic metals interferes with pyruvic acid levels, which impairs the energy supply to brain cells. In young children this would be of particular significance since, up to age four, children experience greater oxygen demand in the brain than adults do. A federal court recently upheld the claims of environmentalists that lead emissions are harmful, and the Environmental Protection Agency has been ordered to add the toxic metal, lead, to its list of air pollutants. (*Wall Street Journal*, Wednesday, March 3, 1976). The greatest, strongest, most immovable forces blocking the improvement of our children's environment in the air we breathe, the food we eat, and the water we drink are the mammoth corporations whose activities continue to impair the environment dangerously.

A report that chronic daily ingestion of lead produced no change in the behavioral pattern of rhesus monkeys was published by the research arm of the lead and zinc industry, despite the fact that experimental evidence favors the view that lead does produce behavioral abnormalities in animals and, more importantly, in man. Moreover, most of mankind appears to be more sensitive than rats and rhesus monkeys to lead. A report in 1960 revealed a high spontaneous abortion rate among female workers in the lead industry. The central barrier does not protect the fetus against the lead to which its mother is exposed.

research

The following sections deal with significant findings in areas relevant to learning disabilities.

HYPOGLYCEMIA

Experimentally induced hypoglycemia, hypoxia (lack of oxygen) and hyperbilirubinemia (jaundice) can produce lesions in newborn experimental animals not unlike those found in mentally retarded children or in those with a history of comparable biochemical disturbances in the perinatal period. The situation is exceedingly complex and controversial in infants with hypoglycemia, many of whom are of low birth weight and have suffered from intrauterine malnutrition. There is good evidence of antenatal brain damage in a significant proportion of these children. Severe symptomatic hypoglycemia rarely occurs on its own, and it is, therefore, not surprising that the lesions found in children or experimental animals dying after hypoglycemic episodes are not specific and are difficult to distinguish from those produced by other causes. Dr. Gerald F. Lucey has reported hypoglycemia in the newborn is much more prevalent than many physicians believe. He stated that anyone not finding 2 to 3 cases per 1,000 live births is probably missing it. He reports the incidence among prematures is 43 per 1,000. A blood sugar level of less than 20 mgs. per 100 ml. in a premature infant or 30 mg. per 100 mg. in a full-term infant is too low. He concludes there is strong evidence hypoglycemia causes brain damage. He cites tremors and cyanosis as early signs of hypoglycemia in the newborn; apnea, apathy, and a high-pitched cry are other early signs. Convulsions are a late sign of hypoglycemia. Dr. Lucey recommends all small-for-birthdate infants should also be checked, as should the large infants of diabetic mothers. He concludes the symptoms of hypoglycemia are caused by a deprivation of glucose in the brain. It reflects inadequate intrauterine nutrition or inadequate glucose homeostasis.

NEUROTRANSMITTERS: DOPAMINE

Administration of 6-hydroxydopamine to neonatal rats produced a rapid and profound depletion of brain dopamine. Total activity of treated animals was signifantly greater than that of controls between 12 and 22 days of age, but then declined, an activity pattern similar to that seen in affected children. This suggests a functional deficiency of brain dopamine in the pathogenesis of minimal brain dysfunction (Shaywitz et al. 1976).

NIACINAMIDE

Niacinamide has been shown to increase rapid eye movement (REM) sleep in mice by 17 percent. In adult human volunteers the administration of 1 gram of niacinamide three times daily increased REM sleep by 40 percent. Several volunteers in this study reported to the author they slept fewer hours and awakened more refreshed during the period they were taking the niacinamide (Beaton *et al.* 1974).

The results of this study show high doses of niacinamide may have behavioral effects unconnected with its role as a vitamin. The best-known drug that increases REM is reserpine, which suggests that further pharmacological study of niacinamide in this light might be of interest. One study (Beaton, in press) reports administration of 250 to 500 mg. per kg. of niacinamide reduced the wheel-running activity in gerbils by 30 percent. The lower dosages of niacinamide, although inducing an initial decrease in activity, were inactive. This report also concludes that niacinamide must have central effects unrelated to its role as a vitamin and the degree to which the therapeutic effects of niacinamide are related to the observed sedative effects are worthy of further investigation.

5-HYDROXYTRYPTOPHAN

Burkhard Scherer and Wolf Kramer (1972) reported that the ability of some niacin compounds to inhibit the tryptophan-pyrrolase or to repress the denovo-synthesis of this enzyme is possibly responsible for the increase of brain 5-hydroxytryptophan by 17 percent after niacinamide administration. The sedation observed at the same time may be due to this 5-HT increase. They concluded: "How far the sedative effects and the repeatedly published therapeutic effects on psychoses can be based on an increased 5-HT formation should be studied by further analysis of the 5-HT turnover. The doses applied by us to rats in any case are far above the doses given to man for therapeutic reasons."

D. J. Boullin and colleagues (1970) were able to report highly singificant abnormalities in platelet 5-HTP efflux in autistic children, as compared to normal controls. In a second study (Boullin *et al.* 1971) the abnormality was found in nearly all cases diagnosed as autistic, but in *no* case diagnosed "psychotic but not autistic." The laboratory work was done without knowledge of the clinical diagnoses.

At the symposium on orthomolecular psychiatry in the First World Congress on Biological Psychiatry which convened in Buenos Aires, in September 1974, the research team of Drs. G. Buyze, W. J. H. Driss, A. J. Schakellar and W. R. P. Schreurs of the Netherlands reported that, according to Linus Pauling's (1968) concept of orthomolecular psychiatry, the treatment of mental illness should benefit by optimalization of the molecular environment of the mind. In this connection, the effect of multiple vitamin administration was studied in 80 hospitalized psychiatric patients divided into two equal groups matched in age, sex, diagnosis, and psychiatric treatment. During the experimental period of three months, treatment and medications were kept constant. One group received a daily vitamin mixture of thiamine, pyridoxine, B-12, nicotinamide, and folic acid of three times the recommended daily allowance (RDA). The second group received placebo. The vitamin blood levels were determined before and after the experimental period. Assessment of the psychiatric effect was made by measurement of the scores with an ego-strength scale and with a social adjustment scale (Beyart 1966). In a number of patients, subnormal or borderline values for one or more of the vitamin concentrations were found. Statistical analysis of the scores in the two rating scales used showed an improvement in the vitamin-supplemented group. Dr. Buyze and colleagues will publish their findings this year in the Congress Proceedings.

PYRIDOXINE

In a study reported in the *Journal of Nutrition and Metabolism* (Lindenbaum and Mueller 1974), the authors reported that vitamin B-6 (pyridoxine) is involved in some way in regulating the glucose levels in the blood of stressed mice, possibly by affecting the levels of the enzyme phosphorylase or by affecting the metabolism of tryptophan in the kynurenine pathway. It also seems that B-6 plays a role in regulating a methylation process that could be related to the production of psychogenic substances, specifically di/methyl/oxy/phenyl/ethylamine. This regulation could come about as a result of the augmentation of the production of nicotinic acid in the kynurenine pathway. Thus, pyridoxine would seem to have a regulatory effect on tryptophan metabolism, but does not appear to affect the production or metabolism of serotonin from tryptophan.

The role played by pyridoxine in the production of norepinephrine is not clear since the effects of elevated levels of glucose (associated with administration of B-6) on the levels of norepinephrine in the brain are uncertain. Finally, a decrease in ulcer formation was noted in the mice receiving B-6 which tends to implicate the vitamin in an antistress role. A study reported to the Canadian Mental Health Association in 1972 described the use of the vitamin pyridoxine (B-6), in the treatment of certain types of schizophrenia and its role in the potentiation of therapeutic effects of nicotinic acid by pyridoxine in chronic schizophrenics (Ananth *et al.* 1972). Other investigators reported that nicotinic acid one of the products of pyridoxine-dependent pathways was useful in the treatment of some psychiatric patients.

drug abuse and juvenile delinquency

When the widespread use of marijuana, the major hallucinogens, and other illicit drugs began in the late 1950s, a correlation was noted in drug use, failing academic performance, and loss of interest in school in able students. The onset of schizophrenia in early adolescence is most often manifested by depression, loss of concentration, impaired attention span and loss of interest which leads to a marked decline in academic performance. These signs are manifest early in the illness and may precede by a year or more the development of the more dramatic perceptual distortions and delusions characteristic of schizophrenia. Similar symptoms may be considered premonitory signs of the first stages of drug abuse in a child.

Because the learning-disabled child is not readily accepted by his peer group, who have over the years labeled him "a retard" or "just stupid" and ridiculed his clumsy ineffectiveness in sports or other group games or activities, he ultimately is brought to the point in his life when he may pay any price to anyone granting acceptance. He happily and willingly becomes a follower of any member of his peer group who accepts him without ridicule or reservation. In the classroom he becomes the clown who makes the other children laugh at his bizarre antics, his foolish talk. His classmates certainly do take notice of him, and the other nonconformists in the school accept him. In my clinical experience, I have found this to be the route by which a large percentage of learning-disabled children drop into the drug culture and juvenile delinquency. I have examined and treated many hundreds of learning-disabled adolescents who began the use of marijuana while in the elementary grades and lost what little interest in learning remained as they were pushed through the grades finally to drop out of school. Many expressed the feeling they had "better things to do than go to school." Too often, the better things they did was to graduate to the use of major hallucinogens like LSD and mescaline. If engaging in regular use of illicit drugs or in actual delinquent behavior such as theft or burglary is the fee to be paid for acceptance, he readily agrees.

When a child decides he is better off out of school, he has made a decision about a lifestyle which will ease the unbearable tension and anxiety which daily attendance coupled with daily failure creates for him. The decision is soon implemented by acts of truancy which in most cases is the precursor to delinquency. Dr. MacDonald Critchley, the British authority in reading and language disorders, found 75 percent of a group of delinquents illiterate. Wherever groups of delinquent children have been surveyed, 60 to 80 percent read below grade level and many aged 18 to 22 could not perform on a fourth grade reading level. In 1967, the U. S. Public Health Service reported 75 percent of delinquent children in New York were illiterate. Howard James is quoted in the book *Something's Wrong with My Child*, a book dealing with the juvenile justice system, that in at least 80 percent of all cases which come to the juvenile courts it can be found that a school problem was an important factor.

A Bureau of Prisons report reveals 90 percent of the inmates of federal prisons have reading problems. Society adds hundreds of thousands of new school dropouts each year to the millions who preceded them to roam our city streets unable to find work because they can't read.

In a report presented to the First World Congress of Biological Psychiatry in Buenos Aires in September, 1974, Dr. Eugene Ziskind, Professor of Psychiatry at UCLA's School of Medicine, reported a study whose major thesis was based on the tendency of sociopaths to undergo spontaneous remission at midlife. Ziskind and his coworkers made the assumption that those sociopaths who do not undergo remission have failed because their pathological behavior has ruined the possibilities of such an outcome. The report continued that their data are consistent with the hypothesis that most sociopaths are the subjects of a lag in behavioral development and stressed that the earliest treatment efforts should be focused on preventing incarceration. Therefore, energetic treatments of disabilities should be made available early in life for those who have symptoms of the minimal brain dysfunction syndrome with specific learning disabilities. Rejection by parents, teachers, and peers must be reduced to the lowest possible minimum by securing adequate understanding for the subject's disability. Suspension from school should be discouraged and school dropouts not permitted. Assessment should be made of the unique patterns of learning of which each subject is capable. Dr. Ziskind described a treatment approach involving a variety of experts whose particular expertise would be to create a constructive climate to prevent or replace "bad company" and criminal contacts. Group therapy, feedback, behavioral therapy, and chemotherapy with psychoactive drugs are also being explored in their multidimensional approach to treatment.

In a thirty-year followup study of 524 child psychiatric patients by Dr. A. P. Derdeyn of the University of Virginia Medical Center, it was found that not a single child developed an antisocial personality as an adult in the absence of anti-social symptoms as a child. Fifty percent of the antisocial children continued their antisocial behavior as adults; of the other half of the adults who had been antisocial as children, 90 percent were exhibiting maladaptive behavior consisting of alcohol addiction, major mental illness, or severe marital or employment problems (1974).

closing statement

A measure of the state of its civilization is any society's attitude toward its handicapped. If we are to continue to count ourselves among the leaders of the civilized world, we must gain a new perspective on the things we do for and to our most precious commodity—our children. We feed them foods containing allowable amounts of filth approved by the FDA. Included in this filth are mouse droppings and animal hair. They eat hot dogs containing allowable amounts of bone splinters and bone dust. All their luncheon meats are treated with sodium nitrite and other additives. Most of their food and beverages contain artificial colors and flavors which produce hyperactivity in a significant percentage of their population and seriously interfere with their ability to learn. We then add to all this the lead and the stench in the air they breathe. From the billions of cigarettes we consume, we blow cadmium, another toxic metal, into their air space. We then punish them for their inability to learn. Only after due consideration of these disasters can we understand the enormity of the problem our children share with us.

appendix

Good nutrition depends on eating a well balanced diet which should consist of modest portions of all foods currently available. Eat fresh, whole foods, try new foods, but keep the meals simple.

Avoid:

> All white flour, refined sugar, salt, coffee, tea, cola beverages, chocolate and foods containing additives, artificial flavors or colors.

Include:

> Raw seeds—sunflower, pumpkin and sesame.
>
> Raw nuts—walnut, pecan, almond, filbert, cashew.
>
> Raw fruits—fresh, unsprayed or washed (do not use canned or frozen).
>
> Raw or steamed vegetables—many vegetables which are usually cooked can be eaten raw in salads, eg., spinach, cauliflower, beets, carrots, peppers, cabbage, onions, bean and seed sprouts. Salads should be eaten every day. Seeds and nuts can be added to salads. Salad dressing

should be fresh and include a variety of cold pressed oils with cider vinegar or fresh lemon juice, garlic and herbs.

Yoghurt—plain, to which you may add fresh fruit or nuts or both. It is best to get acidophilus cultured yoghurts.

Cheeses—may be eaten in moderation and can include cottage cheese, cheddar, swiss and any natural unprocessed cheese.

Eggs—it is good to include some eggs in the diet although it is not absolutely necessary.

Whole grains and legumes—rice, millet, oats, barley, rye, wheat, beans (including soybeans).

All small fish like trout, flounder. Avoid large fish like swordfish: small fish accumulate much less mercury.

SUGGESTED MENU

BREAKFAST—medium orange or grapefruit or fruit, or juice, one egg; only one slice of bread or toast with butter; beverage.

LUNCH— meat, cheese, or fish; salad (large serving of lettuce, tomato, or salad with mayonnaise or French dressing); vegetables; two slices of bread or toast; dessert; beverage.

SUGGESTED SNACKS—glass of milk or juice, nuts, seeds, fruit, cheese, pickles, carrot sticks, celery sticks (plain or stuffed with cream cheese), yoghurt.

DINNER—soup, if desired (not thickened with flour); vegetables; liberal portion of lean meat, fish, or poultry; one slice only of bread, if desired; dessert; milk.

BEFORE BEDTIME—juice or nuts, if desired.

RECOMMENDED FOODS

ALLOWABLE VEGETABLES—asparagus, avocado, beets, broccoli, brussel sprouts, cabbage, carrots, cauliflower, celery, cucumber, eggplant, lima beans, onions, radishes, sauerkraut, squash, stringbeans, tomatoes, turnips, green peas, artichokes.

ALLOWABLE FRUITS—apricots, berries, grapefruit, melons, oranges, peaches, pears, pineapple, tangerines. May be raw or cooked, with or without cream, but without sugar. Canned fruits must be without sugar.

JUICE—any unsweetened fruit or vegetable juice, except grape juice or prune juice. For example, apple, grape-fruit, orange, pineapple, carrot, tomato, apricot or cranberry (without sugar).

DESSERTS—unsweetened gelatin, dried, raw or cooked fruit with or without whipped cream (whipped cream must be homemade without sugar), cheese, fresh fruit, apple-sauce, honey dipped apples, fruit stuffed with nuts and seeds, melon baskets, fresh fruit salad, fruit parfaits, topped with chopped nuts and unsweetened coconut, cold or hot carob milk (with or without homemade whipped cream), frozen "juice pops," frozen juice and yoghurt mix.

SMALL AMOUNTS—potatoes, rice, corn, grapes, raisins, plums, figs, dates, bananas, prunes, spaghetti, macaroni, noodles. (If spaghetti, macaroni or noodles are served, do not serve bread with that meal.)

EVEN SMALLER AMOUNTS OF—the following only if made without sugar (honey may be used): pie, cookies, cake, pastries, sweet custards, puddings, ice cream (ice cream sweetened with honey and sugarless honey graham crackers are available on the market). If honey is used for sweetener, not more than one teaspoonful daily.

AVOID COMPLETELY—cane sugar and any derivative and
all products made with sugar, date sugar, caffeine-
ordinary coffee, strong brewed tea, cola beverages and
all sodas.

SALICYLATE-FREE DIET

These foods and products should be avoided.

FOODS

Almonds	Nectarines
Apples	Oranges
Apricots	Peaches
Blackberries	Plums or prunes
Cherries	Raspberries
Currants	Strawberries
Gooseberries	Cucumbers and pickles
Grapes or raisins	Tomatoes

FLAVORINGS (Omit artificial flavors and colors in foods and drinks)

Ice Cream	Cloves
Oleomargarine	Oil of wintergreen
Gin and all distilled bev-verages (except vodka)	Toothpaste and tooth-power
Cake mixes	Mint flavors
Bakery goods (except plain bread)	Mouthwash
Jello	Jam or jelly
Candies	Luncheon meats (salami, bologna, etc.)
Gum	Frankfurters (hot dogs)

BEVERAGES

Cider and cider vinegars	Gin and all distilled drinks (except vodka)
Wine and wine vinegars	
Powdered, artificially flavored beverages	All tea
	Beer
Soda pop (all soft drinks)	Diet drinks and supplements

DRUGS AND MISCELLANEOUS

All medicines containing aspirin (i.e., most available home cold remedies).

Perfumes.

Toothpaste and toothpowder (a mixture of salt and soda, or unscented hypoallergenic soap, can be used as a substitute).

Note: Check all labels of prepared foods or drugs for artificial flavoring and artificial coloring.

FOODS HIGH IN ESSENTIAL NUTRIENTS

MAGNESIUM
Soy flour
Whole wheat
Oatmeal
Peas
Brown rice
Whole corn
Beans
Nuts
Wheat germ
Cocoa

SODIUM
The greatest portion of sodium is provided by table salt and salt used in cooking. Foods high in sodium include:
Dried beef
Ham
Canned corned beef
Bacon
Wheat breads
Salted crackers
Flaked breakfast cereals

PHOSPHORUS
Highest dietary sources include protein foods such as:
Soy flour
Whole wheat
Oatmeal
Peas
Brown rice
Whole corn
Beans
Nuts

CALCIUM
Cheese
Milk
Bread
Nuts
Legumes
Green leafy vegetables

Olives
Cheese
Butter
Margarine
Sausage
Dried fish
Canned vegetables
Shellfish and salt water fish
Raw celery

VITAMIN B-1
Liver
Pork
Yeast
Organ meats
Whole grains
Bread
Wheat germ
Peanuts

VITAMIN C
Citrus
Fresh fruits
Berries
Broccoli
Tomatoes
Green leafy vegetables
Baked potatoes
Turnips

PANTOTHENIC ACID
Liver
Organ meats
Eggs
Yeast

IRON
Liver
Organ meats
Eggs
Legumes
Green leafy vegetables
Oysters

POTASSIUM
Green leafy vegetables
Legumes
Nuts
Cocoa
Vegetable juice

VITAMIN B-2
Eggs
Liver
Yeast
Milk
Whole grains
Bread
Wheat germ

NIACIN
Yeast
Liver
Whole bran
Peanuts
Beans

VITAMIN B-6
Wheat germ
Kidney
Liver
Ham

Wheat bran
Legumes
Cereals

VITAMIN E
Margarine
Oil salad dressing
Vegetable oils
Eggs
Cereal germ

VITAMIN A
Carrots
Green leafy vegetables
Butter
Whole milk
Liver
Fish

PROTEIN
Eggs
Milk
Cheese
Fish
Chicken
Beef
Pork
Soybeans
Beans
Peas
Nuts

FATS
Margarine
Butter
Peanut butter

Organ meats
Legumes
Peanuts

IODINE
Iodized salt
Shellfish
Ocean fish
Bacon

VITAMIN B-12
Liver
Organ meats
Oysters
Salmon
Eggs
Beef

AMINO ACIDS
Soy milk
Fish
Beef
Soy flour
Organ meats
Shellfish
Eggs
Milk
Whole wheat
Liver
Cheese

POLYUNSATURATED
FATTY ACIDS
Margarine from safflower,
    corn, soy (non hydro-
    genated)
Corn oil (35%)

Salad oils	Safflower oil (70%)
Cream	Peanut oil (28%)
Cheese	Soybean oil (50%)
Bacon	Cottonseed oil (50%)
Pork	Lard (10%)
Beef	
Fish	

COMMON FOODS WITH HIGH CONCENTRATIONS OF TRACE MINERALS

IRON	COPPER
Beef juice	Calf liver
Hog liver	Oysters
Parsley	Beef liver
Beef liver	Molasses
Molasses	Mushrooms
Egg yolk	Pecans
Sweetbreads	Peanuts
Raisins	Walnuts
Watercress	Pickles
Avocado	Lobsters
Bran flakes	Rice
Dates	Bran flakes
Wheat	Olives
Beef	Nuts
Oatmeal	Cereals
Pickles	Fruits
Spinach	Leafy vegetables
Mushrooms	Meat
Oysters	Brewer's yeast
Reinforced foods (bread,	Lobster
breakfast cereal, or flour)	Molasses
Leafy vegetables	
Nuts	
Cereals	

Meats
Tubers
Fruits
Brewer's yeast

IODINE
Cod liver oil
Sea foods
Agar
Eggs
Oats
Peaches
Butter
Lamb
Applesauce
Bread
Celery
Asparagus
Bananas
Beef
Lemons
Olive oil
Canned pears
Potatoes
Cottage cheese
Cream '
Spinach
Corn
Fresh water fish

SODIUM
Butter
Cheese
Clams
Oysters
Bread

MANGANESE
Wheat bran
Blueberries
Huckleberries
Pecans ·
Graham bread
Oatmeal
Walnuts
Barley
Peanuts
Cocoanut
Rye bread
Beets
Bananas
Lettuce
Parsley
Oatflakes
Cocoa
Buckwheat flour
Split peas, dried
Walnuts
Peanuts
Turnip greens

ZINC
Oysters
Commercial casein
Cereals
Fruits
Meat
Vegetables
Cow's milk

Egg white
Celery
Olives
Raisins
Beets
Beef
Spinach
Carrots
Cauliflower
Oatmeal
Pumpkin
Turnips
Broccoli
Melons
Egg yolk
Milk
Peanuts

CALCIUM
Cream cheese
Egg yolk
Broccoli
Cow's milk
Cauliflower
Cream
Chocolate
Pecans
Walnuts
Cottage cheese
Spinach
Bran flakes
Celery
Eggs
Peanuts
Oatmeal
Raisins

POTASSIUM
Olives
Molasses
Raisins
Peanuts
Parsnips
Spinach
Wheat
Potatoes
Rye
Broccoli
Oatmeal
Sweet potato
Banana
Mushrooms
Beets
Turnips
Pumpkin
Carrots
Cocoanuts
Figs

CHLORIDE
Butter
Clams
Rye bread
Cheese
Oysters
Graham crackers
Bread
Molasses
Celery
Egg white
Bananas
Cocoanut
Eggs

Turnips
Beans (cooked)
Oysters
Wheat
Breast milk
Sardines
Molasses
Turnip greens
Salmon
Yoghurt

MAGNESIUM
Peanuts
Pecans
Walnuts
Oatmeal
Clams
Raisins
Spinach
Wheat germ
Cocoa
Cashew nuts
Almonds
Soybeans
Brazil nuts
Split peas, dried
Whole grain rice
(Dairy products, fruits,
    and vegetables have
    low concentrations)

Milk
Egg yolk
Sweet potato
Cream
Raisins
Beef
Lettuce
Spinach
Oatmeal

TOTAL PHOSPHATE (AS PHOSPHORUS)
Cheese
Egg yolk
Bran flakes
Yeast
Oatmeal
Puffed wheat
Peanuts
Wheat
Walnuts
Pecans
Shredded Wheat
Ham
Cottage cheese
Whole wheat bread
Fish
Turkey
Eggs
Liver
Pork
Chicken
Lamb
Lobster
Beef

SODIUM (Na) AND POTASSIUM (K) IN COMMON FOODS

Food	Mineral content Na mg%	K mg%
Nuts		
Almonds	2.0	690
Brazil nuts	0.8	650
Filberts	0.8	560
Peanuts (unsalted)	0.8	740
Walnuts	2.0	450
Fruits		
Apples	0.1	68
Apricots	0.5	440
Bananas	0.1	400
Cherries	1.0	280
Lemons	0.6	130
Oranges	0.2	170
Peaches	0.1	180
Plums	0.1	140
Strawberries	0.7	180
Cereals		
Barley	3.0	160
Corn	0.4	290
Oats	2.0	340
Rice	0.8	100
Legumes		
Beans, in pod	0.8	300
Lima beans, fresh	1.0	700
Navy beans, dry	0.9	1300
Peas, fresh	0.9	380
Green leafy vegetables (edible portion)		
Broccoli	16.0	400
Cabbage	5.0	230
Cauliflower	24.0	400

Lettuce	12.0	140
Spinach	190.0	790
Celery stalks	110.0	300
Root vegetables (less skins)		
Beets	110.0	350
Carrots	31.0	410
Potatoes	0.6	410
Turnips (yellow)	5.0	260
Hen's eggs		
Whole egg (less shell)	140.0	130
Milk and milk products		
Human milk	40.0	64
Cow's milk	51.0	140
Butter (unsalted)	5.0	4
Butter (salted)	980.0	––
Cheese (cheddar)	540.0	130
Cheese (cottage)	320.0	80
Meats and fish (less bone and excess fat)		
Beef	53.0	380
Chicken leg	110.0	250
Cod	60.0	360
Calf liver	110.0	380
Lamb	110.0	340
Pork	58.0	260
Turkey leg	92.0	310

ADDITIVES

Foods containing the following additives should be avoided:

Sodium nitrite	Sodium benzoate
Gum arabic	Disodium EDTA
Saccharin	Butylated hydroxyanisole
Sodium acid pyrophosphate	(BHA)

FDC red No. 2
FDC yellow No. 5
Monosodium glutamate
Heptyl paraben
Sodium propionate

Butylated hydroxytoluene
  (BHT)
Brominated vegetable oil
All artificial flavors
All artificial colors

LEAD SOURCES

This listing of 60 sources of lead has been documented from the literature of the world:

Airplane exhausts
Alloys
Asphalt
Auto exhaust fumes
Auto heaters
Auto air conditioners
Batteries
Building debris
Bones of animals; bone meal
Cement dust
Ceramic materials
Charcoal
Coal gas
Cosmetics
Crops
Dolomite
Dust
Dyes
Fertilizers
Foods
Furnace burners
Gas burners
Gasoline
Glass (leaded)
Some hair shampoos, hair
  rinses, hair sprays

Oils, petroleum, crude
Paints
Paint on pencils
Pesticides
Pewter ware
Plaster
Poultry
Print shops
Printed paper
Putty
Rain
Road dust
Roots, crops
Rubber, tires
Scrap metals
Smelters
Smogs
Smoke
Snow
Solder
Soils
Tobacco
Toys
Trees (forest fires)
Vegetables
Water

Incinerators
Linotype
Meats
Minerals (crude)
Newsprint

Water condensed
  from dehumidifiers
Water pipes
Welding
Some wines

glossary

ALA dehydratase—an enzyme present in the brain. Its normal activity is inhibited by the presence of lead in the body.

amino acids—structural units of protein. Of the 22 amino acids, 8 are called "essential," since our bodies cannot make these. The "essential" amino acids are leucine, isoleucine, lysine, methionine, phenylalanine, tryptophan, threonine, and valine.

amphetamine—stimulant drug used to control hyperactivity.

anemia—condition in which the blood is deficient in red cells or iron.

autism—a developmental disorder manifesting itself within the first few months of life and characterized by aloof, withdrawn personality that causes children to appear isolated and living in a private inaccessible dream world. Within the first two years of development, disturbed behavior such as prolonged rocking, head banging, disinterest in surroundings, unusual fear of strangers, obsessive interest in certain toys or mechanical appliances, tense, repetitive ritualistic behavior, and insistence on the preservation of sameness in the environment develop. Child develops either nonverbally or, if he does have speech, is unable to use language as a means of communication.

beriberi—an illness produced by a deficiency of thiamine (vitamin B-1).

calcium pantothenate—the calcium salt of pantothenic acid, one of the B-complex vitamins.

catecholamines—norepinephrine, dopamine, and serotonin; catecholamines are generally regarded as neurotransmitters.

chelate—lead or other heavy metals are removed from the tissues by the use of a medication called a chelating agent. Such medications combine with the heavy metals in the tissues and form a new compound which is soluable and which the body can then discharge. The word is derived from the Greek *chela*, meaning "claw."

dopamine—a catecholamine, a substance formed in the brain.

dopamine metabolite homovanillic acid—chemical produced during the metabolism of dopamine. Levels of homovanillic acid can be measured in the cerebrospinal fluid and are taken as reflections of the activity of the neurons in the brain in which dopamine is formed.

dyslexia—difficulty in learning to read despite conventional instruction, adequate intelligence and sociocultural opportunities.

electroencephalogram (EEG)—brain wave tracing.

folic acid—one of the B-complex vitamins; it is involved in the formation of RNA and DNA and is fundamental in cell division and growth.

general learning disability (GLD)—term used to describe the problems of those children who have difficulty learning anything. This condition occurs in children who grow up with some severe developmental disorder such as autism, childhood schizophrenia, brain damage, or mental retardation.

hydroxytryptophan—tryptophan combines with an enzyme to form 5-hydroxytryptophan. 5-hydroxytryptophan is then converted to serotonin, a neurotransmitter.

hyperactivity—excessive movement which the child cannot control. See *hyperkinesis.*

hyperinsulinism—excessive amount of insulin in the bloodstream.

hyperkinesis—technical term for hyperactivity; literally "excessive movement."

hypoglycemia—condition produced by an insufficient amount of glucose (sugar) in the bloodstream. Commonly known as low blood sugar.

insulin—hormone produced by the pancreas. Lack of sufficient insulin results in diabetes.

learning disability (LD)—term used to describe the problems of those children who are not mentally retarded but who have difficulty learning due to subtle central nervous system dysfunctions. Such children do not exhibit gross psychological or sensory impairment.

megavitamin—any vitamin used in doses many times larger than its Recommended Daily Allowance dose.

methylphenidate—generic name of Ritalin, a stimulant, the most widely used drug to control hyperactive behavior.

minimal brain dysfunction (MBD)—term used to describe the problems of those children whose symptomatology appears in one or more of the specific areas of brain function, but in mild or subclinical form without reducing overall intellectual functioning to subnormal ranges.

neuroleptics—drugs which are active in the central nervous system and which influence behavior, perception, thought and mood.

neurotransmitters—substances formed in the brain which transmit electrical impulses from one brain cell to the next of the trillions of cells in the brain.

niacin—nicotinic acid, a form of vitamin B-3. It is a constituent of nicotinamide adenodinucleotide (NAD).

niacinamide—a form of vitamin B-3.

nicotinamide adenodinucleotide (NAD)—a coenzyme formed in the body from nicotinic acid.

norepinephrine—a catecholamine; a substance formed in the brain.

orthomolecular therapy—treatment based on the principle of raising to proper levels of concentration those substances normally present in the body.

pellagra—an illness caused by deficiency of niacin in the diet.

placebo—substitute for a medication; an inert substance that cannot benefit a patient.

pharmacotherapy—treatment or healing with the use of drugs.

psychotropic drugs—drugs commonly known as tranquilizers. See *neuroleptics.*

pyridoxine—vitamin B-6.

REM sleep—one of the normal stages of sleep characterized by rapid eye movement (REM).

riboflavin—vitamin B-2.

salicylate—product derived from coal tar.

schizophrenia—an illness characterized by perceptual distortions, disorder in thinking, disturbed behavior, and depression. Childhood schizophrenia is very frequently difficult to distinguish from autism, but the schizophrenic child generally does not manifest the insistence on preservation of sameness, the aloofness, or the severe disturbance of speech development. Childhood schizophrenia very often will not be overtly manifested during the first few years of life.

scurvy—an illness produced by a deficiency of vitamin C.

Snellen Chart—standard eye chart used to test for sight.

sociopath—one who manifests extreme antisocial behavior.

specific learning disabilities (SLD)—term used to describe the problems of those children who have difficulty learning specific subjects such as reading and math.

therapy—that branch of medicine concerned with the remedial treatment of disease; it may also be defined as the art of healing.

tryptophan—one of the essential amino acids; present in protein foods. It is the dietary precursor of serotonin.

references

Ananth, J.V., Ban, T.A., Lehmann, H.E. and Bennett, J. 1970. Nicotinic acid in the prevention and treatment of Methionine induced
exacerbation of psychopathology in schizophrenics. *Journal of
Canadian Psychiatric Association* 15:15.

Beaton, J.M., Pegram, G.V., Smythies, J.R. and Bradley, R.J. 1974.
Niacinamide. *Separatum Experientia* 30, p. 926.

Boullin, D.J., Coleman, M. and O'Brien, R.A. 1970. Abnormalities in
platelet 5-hydroxytryptamine efflux in patients with infantile
autism. *Nature* 226, p. 371.

Boullin, D.J., Coleman, M., O'Brien, R.A. and Rimland, B. 1971. Laboratory predictions of infantile autism based on 5-hydroxytryp-
tamine efflux from blood platelets and their correlation with the
Rimland E-2 Score. *Journal of Autism and Childhood Schizophrenia* 1:1, pp 63-71.

Bronfenbrenner, U. 1969. Dampening the unemployability explosion.
Saturday Review 4 January 1969.

Brutten, M., Richardson, S.O. and Mangel, C. 1973. *Something's wrong
with my child.* New York: Harcourt Brace Jovanovich.

Bryce-Smith, D. and Waldron, H.A. 1974. Lead pollution, disease and
behavior. *Community Health* 6: 1968.

Bryce-Smith, D. 1971. Lead poisoning. *Chemistry in Britain* 7:54.

Caprio, R.J., Margulis, H.L. and Joselow, M.M. 1974. Lead absorption in children and its relationship to urban traffic densities. *Archives of Environmental Health* 28, pp. 195-197.

Cott, A. 1971. Orthomuscular approach to the treatment of learning disabilities. *Schizophrenia* 3:2, pp.95-105.

Cott, A. 1972. Megavitamins: the orthomuscular approach to behavioral disorders and learning disabilities. *Academic Therapy* 7:3, pp. 245-258.

David, O.J. *et al.* 1976. Lead and hyperactivity:behavioral response to chelation. *American Journal of Psychiatry* 113:10, pp. 1155-1158.

Derdeyn, A.P. 1974. Personality development and personality disorders, with emphasis on anti-social personality. *Psychiatry Digest* 10, p. 28.

Dohan, F.C., Grasberger, J.C., Lowell, F.M., Johnston, H.T. and Arbegast, A.W. 1969. Relapsed schizophrenics: more rapid improvement on a milk-and-cereal diet. *The British Journal of Psychiatry* 115, p. 522.

Hamilton, A. and Hardy, H.L. 1949. Industrial toxicology. Paul B. Hoeber. pp. 94-103.

Hoffman, M.S. 1971. Early indications of learning problems. *Academic Therapy* 7:1, pp. 23-35.

Kasowski, M.A. and Kasowski, W.J. 1976. The burden of lead: how much is safe? *CMA Journal* 114:573.

Lindenbaum, E.S. and Mueller, J.J. 1974. Effects of pyridoxine on mice after immobilization stress. *Journal of Nutrition and Metabolism* 17, pp. 368-374.

Michaelson, I.A. and Sauderhoff, M.W. 1973. Lead poisoning. *Medical World News,* 7 September 1973.

Millar, J.A. *et al.* 1970. Lead and d'Aminolevulinic acid dehydratase levels in mentally retarded children and in lead poisoned suckling rats. *Lancet* 2, pp. 695-698.

Montagu, Ashley. 1964. *Life before birth.* New York: New American Library.

Pasamanick, B. and Kawi, A.A. 1968. Association of factors of pregnancy with reading disorders in childhood. *Journal of the American Medical Association* 22 March 1968, pp. 1420-1423.

Pasamanick, B., Rogers, M.E. and Lilienfeld, A.M. 1956. Pregnancy experience and development of behavior disorders in children. *American Journal of Psychiatry* 112, pp. 613-618.

Pauling, Linus. 1968. Orthomolecular psychiatry. *Science* 1968, pp. 169-256.

Pfeiffer, C.C., *et al.* 1971. A longitudinal study of trace metal therapy in copper loaded schizophrenia patients. *Abstracts of the Annual Meeting for Biological Psychiatry*, 1 May 1971.

Pfeiffer, C.C. 1974. Observations on trace and toxic elements in hair and serum. *Journal of Orthomolecular Psychiatry* 3:4, pp. 259-264.

Rimland, B. 1971. High dosage level of certain vitamins in the treatment of children with severe mental disorders. In *Orthomolecular Psychiatry*, eds. L. Pauling and D. Hawkins. San Francisco: W.H. Freeman Co.

Scherer, B. and Kramer, W. 1972. Influence of niacinamide administration on brain 5-HT and a possible mode of action. *Life Science* 1, pp. 189-195.

Shaywitz, B.A. 1976. Selective brain dopamine depletion in developing rats: an experimental model of minimal brain dysfunction. *Science* 191, pp. 305-308.

Silbergeld, E.K. and Goldberg, A.M. 1973. Effects of lead ingestion on mouse behavior. *Medical World News*, 7 September 1973.

Singh, M.M. and Kay, S.R. 1976. Wheat gluten: a pathogenic factor in schizophrenia. *Science* 191, pp. 401.

Warburg, O. 1966. The prime cause and prevention of cancer. 1966 Lindau Lecture, presented for the Nobel Peace Committee.

Wendle, W.F., Faro, M.D., Barker, J.N., Barsky, D. and Guteirrez, S. 1971. Developmental behaviors: delayed appearance in monkeys asphyxiated at birth. *Science* 171:3976, pp. 1173-1175.

Williams, R.J., Heffley, J.D. and Bode, C.W. 1971. The nutritive value of single foods. Paper presented to the National Academy of Sciences, 28 April 1971.

Wunderlich, R.C. 1970. *Kids, brains and learning.* St. Petersburg, Florida: Johnny Reads, Inc.

Wurtman, R.J. 1975. Nutrition and the brain. *Journal of Food Technology,* March 1975.

Yaryura-Tobias, J. and Neziroglu, B.A. 1975. Violent behavior, brain dysrhythmia and glucose dysfunction. *Journal of Orthomolecular Psychiatry* 4:3, pp. 182-188.

Learning disorders in children (Proceedings of the World Federation of Neurology meeting in Dallas, Texas, 1968, ed. Lester Tarnopol.) New York: Little, Brown.

A list of articles on nutrition and learning disabilities:

Buckley, R.E. 1977. Nutrition, metabolism, brain functions and learning. *Academic Therapy* 12:3, pp. 321-326.

Hawley, C. and Buckley, R.E. 1974. Food dyes and hyperkinetic children. *Academic Therapy* 10:1, pp. 27-32.

Jani, S.N. and Jani, L.A. 1974. Nutritional deprivation and learning disabilities—an appraisal. *Academic Therapy* 11:1, pp. 151-158.

Kronick, Doreen. 1975 Learning from living: a case history—sugar, fried oysters and zinc. *Academic Therapy* aa:a, pp. 119-121.

Krippner, Stanley. 1975. An alternative to drug treatment for hyperactive children. *Academic Therapy* 10:4, pp. 433-439.

Powers, H.W.S., Jr. 1973. Dietary measures to improve behavior and achievement. *Academic Therapy* 9:3, pp. 203-214.

Powers, H.W.S., Jr. 1975. Caffeine, behavior and the LD child. *Academic Therapy* 11:1, p. 5-11.

Wunderlich, R.C. 1973. Treatment of the hyperactive child. *Academic Therapy* 8:4, pp. 375-390.

Wunderlich, R.C. 1975. Biosocial factors in the child with school problems. *Academic Therapy* 10:4, pp. 389-399.